M000235714

QuickStart Keto Diet Guidebook for Beginners

Psychology, Tips & Tricks, And Shortcuts to Start Smoothly.

2-Week Meal Plan Included

By

Anna Lor

Table of Content

Introduction

If you decided to pour a few extra pounds out, you could have encountered a ketogenic diet, which is popularly called the Keto diet. The weight loss plan is common and promises substantial weight loss in a short period of time.

However, far from what most people think the diet is not a magical instrument for losing weight. Just like every other diet, it takes time to adapt and monitor the effects.

The keto diet is meant for the ketosis of your body. This diet is typically low in carbs with high intakes of healthy fats, vegetables and enough proteins. There is also an emphasis on this diet on the avoidance of highly refined foods and sugars.

Keto diets are available in different types: regular cyclical, ketogenic, targeted and high protein diets. The disparity depends on the consumption of carb. The regular ketogenic diet is low in carbs, high in fat, and ample protein.

Most Keto diet critics say that the focus on eating high-fat content is not healthy. This is motivated by the misunderstanding that fats are bad for you. In fact, healthy fats are perfect for you instead.

You can obtain tons of good fats from this diet, such as palm oil, nuts, avocado, fish, eggs, butter, coconut oil, seeds like chia or red meat.

So how does your keto diet work and motivate your body to lose excess pounds? When you have a high-carb diet, the body uses carbohydrate glucose and sugar to fuel your body. When you are on the ketogenic diet, a body is fed limited carbohydrates and sugar.

With reduced sugar and carbohydrates, the glucose levels in the body are exhausted, leading to alternate sources of energy in the body.

This state is known ketosis when the body burns fats for energy other than carbohydrates. When the body gets ketosis, it creates ketones instead of glucose as the source of food. The only two sources of power that drive the brain are ketones and glucose.

Besides only helping to lose weight, putting the body in ketosis often has some health benefits.

The Ketogenic diet is one of the safest diets for weight loss and health enhancement. The diet can also be used for overweight children. Many studies endorse the diet with substantial results.

Chapter 1: Are You Right for The Keto Diet?

Nowadays, it is like everybody is talking about the ketogenic diet, the deficient carb, moderate protein, the fatty diet that turns the body into a fat-burning device. Professional athletes and Hollywood stars openly advocate the benefits of the diet from weight loss, blood sugar reduction, inflammation battle, cancer risk reduction, energy increase and aging slow down. But is keto something you should consider? The following will clarify what this diet is about, the benefits, the drawbacks and the issues.

Normally, glucose is the body's primary energy source. If you eat very small quantities of carbohydrates with only limited amounts of protein (excess protein can be converted to carbohydrates), the body changes its fuel supply to fat much of the time. The liver produces fatty ketones (a fatty acid type). These ketones are a source of fuel for the body, especially for the brain that absorbs a lot of energy and can either be glucose or ketones.

If the body produces ketones, it is metabolically known as ketosis. The best way to reach ketosis is too quickly. If you fast or eat a few carbs and just moderate quantities of protein, your body becomes burning stored fat for fuel. This is why the keto diet appears to lose more weight.

Keto nutrition is not new. It was firstly used in the 1920s as medical treatment to treat epilepsy in infants, but until recently, when anti-epileptic medications appeared on the market, the diet had fallen into obscurity. Owing to the success of the reduction of seizures in epileptic patients, the ability of a diet to treat a variety of neurological conditions and other forms of chronic disease is being studied more and more.

- Neurodegenerative disorders. It can also protect against trauma and stroke in the brain. Keto's neuroprotective effects are based on one hypothesis that ketones produced during ketosis provide brain cells with additional fuel to help these cells resist inflammation damage caused by these illnesses.

- Diabetes and loss of weight. If you try to lose weight, keto diet is successful incredibly as it helps to access and extract the fat from the body. The biggest problem is constant hunger when you try to lose weight. The keto diet aims to prevent this because of the reduction of carbohydrates, and fat intakes encourage satiety and make sticking to the diet more manageable. In the study, obese test lost double their weight on the low-carb (20.7 lbs) diet in 24 weeks compared to a low-fat (10.5 kg) diet.

- Diabetes type 2. Also, to weight loss, a keto diet also tends to increase the response to insulin, which is suitable for people with type 2 diabetes. Researchers have found that diabetics that ate low-carb keto diets could minimize dependency on diabetes medication and eventually even reverse it in a study published in Nutrition & Metabolism. It also enhances other health indicators such as lowering triglyceride and LDL (bad) cholesterol and increasing HDL (good) cholesterol.

- Cancer. Many people do not know that glucose is the critical fuel of cancer cells. This means that eating the right diet will help reduce the development of cancer. Since the keto diet is deficient in carbohydrates, sugar is their primary fuel source for cancer cells. When the body makes ketones, healthy cells will use this as sugar, not cancer cells, so that they are hungry. Studies of keto diets already showed decreased tumor growth and increased survival for a variety of cancers in 1987.

Comparing American Standard, Paleo, and Keto Diets

(As a percentage of the overall calorie consumption)

The main difference among the keto diet and Paleo or American Traditional diets that contains much lower carbohydrates and much fat. The keto diet contributes to ketosis with ketones of 0.5 to 5.0 mm. This can be assessed with a home blood ketone monitor and ketone checks. (Please be conscious that urinary ketones are not correctly tested.)

How to Formulate a Chemical Diet?

1. Carbohydrates Carbsates

For most people, ketosis (getting ketones over 0.5 mm) demands that they limit the number of carbs to about 20-50 grams (g) per day. The exact amount of carbs varies from individual to individual. In general, the more resistant an organism is to insulin, the more resistant it is to ketosis. Some vigorously-trained insulin-sensitive athletes can eat more than 50 g per day and also stay in the ketosis, whereas some people with type 2 diabetes and insulin resistance may need to be close to 20-30 g / day.

Carbs are measured using net biomass, which means total carbs minus fiber and sugar alcohols. The definition of net carbs only includes blood sugar and insulin-enhancing carbohydrates. Fiber has no metabolic or hormonal effect, and most sugar alcohols have no such effect. The exception is maltitol, which can affect sugar and insulin in blood without insignificant impact. Therefore, sugar alcohol should not be excluded from the total carbohydrates if maltitol is on the ingredient list.

The levels of carbs that can and will stay in ketosis can also vary over time, depending on the keto modification, weight loss, practice habits, drugs, etc. Therefore, the ketone levels should be calculated on a regular basis.

Carb-dense foods such as pasta, cereals, potatoes, rice, breasts, candy, sodas, juices and beer are not appropriate for the overall diet.

Most dairy products contain lactose (milk sugar) carbohydrates. Some, however, have fewer carbs and can be used daily. These include hard cheeses (Parmesan, cheddar), mild, high fat (Brie) cheeses, whipped cream, and sour cream.

In general, a carb level below 50 g / day breaks down to the following:

- 5-10 g of protein-based food carbs. Some few remaining grams of natural sources and marinades and additives are applied to the eggs, cheese and shellfish.
- 10-15 g of non-starchy carbohydrates.

- 5-10 g of nut/seed carbs. Most nuts have 5-6 g per ounce of carbs.
- 5-10 g of fruit carbs, including olives, strawberries, avocados and tomatoes.
- 5-10 g of carbs dioxide from a number of sources, such as low carbs sweets, fat dressings or very small sugar beverages.

Having Drinks

Most people want a total fluid of at least half a gallon every day. Filtered water, organic coffee and tea (regular and decaf, unsweetened), unsweetened almond and coconut milk are the best sources. Dietary beverages and sodas are best avoided because they contain artificial sweeteners. When you drink red or white wine, limit the dryer to 1-2 cups. Stop sweetened blended beverages when you drink liquor.

2. Protein

A keto diet is not a diet with high protein. The explanation is that protein raises insulin through a method called gluconeogenesis, thereby inhibiting ketosis, which can be converted into glucose. However, the keto diet must not be too low as it should result in loss of muscle tissue and function.

The average adult needs around 0.8-1.5 g of lean body weight a day per kilogram (kg). The measurement based on lean body weight is essential, not total body weight. The explanation is that fat mass requires no protein to retain, only the slender muscle mass.

The protein requirement will range from 44 (= 54,55 x 0,8) to 82 (= 54,55 x 1,5) g / day if, for example, the body weights 150 lbs (or 150/2.2 = 68,18 kg), and the body fat content is 20 percent (or lean body mass 80% = 68,18 kg by 0.8 = 54,55) g / day.

Those who, for medicinal purposes, avoid insulin or keto diet (cancer, epilepsy, etc.) should be closer to the lower protein limit. For those who are really healthy or athletic, the maximum limit is. The amount of daily protein will lie anywhere between someone else who uses the keto diet for weight loss or other health benefits.

High-quality protein sources include:

8

- Bio-fed eggs (6-8 g of protein/egg)
- Food grass (6-9 g protein/oz)
- Animal sources of omega-3 fats, such as sardines, salmon, and anchovies and herrings from the Alaskan wild catch. (Protein / oz 6-9 g)
- Macadamia, flax, pecans, almonds, sesame and seeds and nuts and seeds. (4-8 g of cup/protein)
- Food (1-2 g protein / oz)

3. Fat

Once the precise amount of carbohydrates and protein to eat has been determined, the remainder of the diet comes from fat. If enough fat is consumed, the weight of the body is preserved. If weight loss is needed, less dietary fat should be eaten, and fat stored for energy use should be used.

For people who eat 2,000 calories a day, daily fat consumption is between 156 and 178 g / day. Fat intakes can reach 300 g / day for large or very active persons with high energy needs to maintain their weight.

Most people can tolerate high-fat intakes, but some circumstances, such as gallbladder removal, can affect fat consumption at a single meal. In this case, more regular meals or bile salts or lipase-high pancreatic enzymes may be beneficial.

No unnecessary fats, such as trans-fat, highly processed multifunctional vegetable oils and large concentrations of multifunctional omega-6, should be consumed.

High-quality fats comprise the best foods:

- Attorneys and Activists Oil
- Cocos and cocoa oil
- Fed butter, ghee and fat of beef
- Strong organic, pastured cream
- Olive oil. Olive oil
- Pastured pig lard
- Triglyceride medium-chain (MCTs)

MCT is a particular fatty form that is metabolized differently from standard long-chain fatty acids. MCTs can be used by the liver to quickly generate energy even before glucose so that ketones are formed.

Concentrated sources of MCT oil as supplements are available. Many people use it to lead to ketosis. Coconut oil is the only food that is special in MCTs. About two-thirds of coconut fat comes from MCT.

Who Does Care For A Keto Diet?

A keto diet is really healthy for most people. However, before such a diet, some people have to take careful care of themselves and talk to their doctors.

- Those who take diabetes drugs. The dosage will have to be modified as blood sugar decreases with a low carbs diet.
- People who take high blood pressure drugs. Dosage can require modification as a low carbs diet reduces blood pressure.
- Shepherds must not eat very strictly, as the body will lose approximately 30 g of carbs per day by milk. Therefore, during breastfeeding, have at least 50 g carbs per day.
- Kidney sufferers should consult their physicians before taking a keto diet.

A Keto Diet General Concerns

- Cannot achieve ketosis. Make sure you do not overeat protein and no secret sugars in the foods you eat.
- Consuming the wrong form of fat like polyunsaturated, highly processed maize and soybean oils.
- "Keto-flu" signs such as lightheadedness, swelling, headaches, exhaustion, brain fog, and constipation. The body appears to excrete more sodium in ketosis. If you don't get enough sodium from your diet, you can develop keto-flu symptoms. It can be quickly remedied by drinking 2 cups of broth per day (with additional salt). You may have to add even more sodium if you exercise intensely or if the sweat rate is high.

- Impact of dawn. Normal blood sugars are lower than 100 mg/dl, and most ketosis patients will reach that if they are not diabetic. In some people, however, blood sugars tend to rise, especially in the morning, while they are on a keto diet. This is the "dawn effect" because of the natural circadian spike in morning cortisol (stress hormone) that causes the liver to produce more glucose. If that happens, make sure that you don't overeat protein at dinner and not too close to bedtime. Stress and inadequate sleep can also contribute to elevated levels of cortisol. If you are immune to insulin, you can also take longer to get ketosis.
- Poor sports results. It usually takes about four weeks for keto-adaptation. During which you turn to something less rigorous instead of performing challenging exercises or preparation. Regular athletic performance back to normal or better after the adaptation time, especially for the endurance sports.
- The Keto-rash is not a recurrent dietary side effect. Probable causes be the development of sweat acetone which irritates skin or the nutrient deficiencies, like minerals and protein. Shower directly after exercise and ensure that all foods are nutrient-dense.
- Cheta-acidosis. This is a very unusual occurrence when blood ketone levels are greater than 15 mm. Ketoacidosis is not caused by a well-developed keto diet. Such conditions such as Type 1 diabetes, SGLT-2 inhibitors or breastfeeding need greater caution. Symptoms include vomiting, nausea, lethargy, and shortness of breath. Sodium bicarbsate, combined with diluted orange or apple juice, can be used to address mild cases. Significant symptoms require urgent medical treatment.

Is Keto Healthy for Long Duration?

This is a contentious area. While no studies have shown that ketosis is a long-term adverse effect, many experts now assume that the human body will develop a 'resistance' to the benefits of ketosis unless it frequently cycles into and out of it. Furthermore, a very high-fat diet may not be sufficient for all body types in the long term.

Cyclical Chinese diet

When you are able to reliably produce over 0.5 mM of ketones in your blood, it is time to reintroduce carbs back into the diet. Instead of only 20-50 g of carbs/day intake, you may want to lift it to 100-150 g during those days. Usually, it would be enough 2-3 times a week. Ideally, this is often achieved on days of strength training, when the protein intake is actually increased.

This cycling method will make the diet scheme more appropriate for some people who are reluctant to remove their favorite food permanently. It can, however, also reduce resistance and adherence to the keto diet or cause binges in sensitive people.

Why Keto Is Actually Good For You

Keto's diets have really been high. It's a perfect way not only to quickly pour those extra pounds but also to remain well. It is more than just a diet for those who have followed the Keto Diet and are still there. It's a way of life, a modern way of life. But as with any significant shift in our lives, it is not easy. It needs unbelievable dedication and determination.

Nice for others, but not for everyone? While the ketogenic diet was used to significantly enhance the quality of life of people, others do not share the thinking of the majority. But why exactly is that? Since we recall that the best way to get rid of the excess weight was to avoid eating the unhealthy foods that we are so used to eating every day. So, to instruct people to eat healthier fats (the main word being more beneficial), you can definitely see why people are suspicious of how and why you are eating more fat to lose weight and do it quickly. This idea goes against all the weight loss we've ever known.

How did Keto begin? -The endocrinologist Rollin Woodrat discovered in 1921 that three water-soluble compounds, B-hydroxybutyrate, Accenture, and Acetoacetate (compound ketone), were formed as a result of malnutrition in the liver or that the person followed a diet rich in high fats and very low carbs. Later that year a man at the Mayo Clinic named Russel Wilder dubbed it "The Ketogenic Diet" and used it with great success to treat epilepsy in young children. But it was substituted because of advances in medicine.

A man named John Struggles Starting Keto-He started Keto on February 2019, had attempted Keto Diet once before six months, but he could never do so for the first week. The first week on Keto was the most challenging part of the whole operation when the feared Keto Flu is also known as carb flu. The Keto flu is a normal reaction to your body as it changes from glucose (sugar) as energy to fat. Many people who go on the Keto Diet claim that it feels like withdrawing from an addictive drug. It can last from 3 days to a whole week. In his case, it lasted just a few days.

People with the keto Flu say they felt drowsy, nauseous, nauseous, dizzy and with terrible migraines. The first week is usually when people want to leave a Keto Diet, note that it happens to everybody early and that the worst part is over when the first week is over. You can use a few treatments to help you resolve this severe spell. Take electrolyte supplements, keep hydrated, drink bone broth, eat more meat, and sleep a lot. Keto Flu is an unfortunate occurrence for all as the body expels the usual regular diet. You've just got to power through.

How do you like a ketogenic diet? If the average person consumes a high-carbs meal, his body takes those carbohydrates and transforms them into fuel glucose. Glucose is the primary source of fuel in the body when carbohydrates are present, when a Keto diet is deficient if any carbohydrates are used, which forces the body to use other kinds of energy so that the body can function well. In the absence of carbohydrates, healthy fats play a part in the liver's taking fatty acids and converting them into ketone bodies.

The perfect Keto diet should be:

- 70 to 80% Fat
- 20-25% protein.
- 5-10% Carbs

You should not consume more than 20 g of carbs a day to sustain the traditional Ketogenic diet. He ate less than 10 g a day for a theatrical experience, but his initial objectives were accomplished, and then some. He lost twenty-eight lbs in a little less than three weeks.

What does ketosis mean? If the body is fully fed, it enters into a "Ketosis" state, which for the body is a normal condition. After the first couple of weeks have been eliminated from the body all the carbohydrates and unhealthy fats, the body is now able to use healthier fats. Ketosis has several potential advantages associated with quick weight loss, health or efficiency. Excessive ketosis can be particularly harmful in some circumstances such as type 1, where, as in some instances, intermittent fasting can be highly effective for people with type 2 diabetes.

What I Can and Can't Eat-It can be really difficult for anyone new to Keto to stick with a low-carb diet, since fat is the cornerstone of this diet. Healthy fats are essential, but you might ask what healthy fat is. Good fat can include grass-fed meats (lamb, goat, beef, and venison), wild fish and seafood, pork and poultry pastures. Salt-free eggs and kinds of butter can also be eaten. Keep away from starchy vegetables, grains, and fruits. Processed foods in no shape or shape are tolerated in the Ketogenic diet, artificial sweetening products and milk can also pose a severe problem.

It's five weeks in and down 34 lbs so far. And feeling fine, he's got massive energy and doesn't crash at work midday as he used to. It will take you seriously and a perfect meal plan to get where you want to be safe. But the route is still more rewarding than where you end up.

Tips for Exercising When on the Ketogenic Diet

When you work out, a lot of things happen. Others are good for your health, and others aren't good – like excessive exercise.

Fitness is a stressor. Although it can be a positive stressor, it can lead to an overdrive of your adrenals. This raises your level of insulin and reduces your ability to lose weight.

When you exercise, your insulin levels increase as your appetite decreases. This also contributes to a substantial drop in the levels of blood sugar, which contributes to hunger.

Although a small rise in insulin levels contributes to a dramatic decrease in fat loss or lipolysis.

One difficulty that we have when we try to lose weight is that we rely too much on the numbers on the scale. We almost unintentionally forget the main factor that loses body fat.

About 80% of our body fat is contained in fat cells. In order to get rid of this accumulated fat, you have to burn it for energy production.

Your body must, however, be in a negative fat balance before it can begin to burn your stored fats for energy. This is a state in which you eat more fat than you do in your diet.

If your body is used to consuming fat to generate energy, both body fat and dietary fat can now be used for energy. This is among the main components of a ketogenic diet for weight loss.

If you do not raise your dietary intake of fat but raise your body's energy by increasing your exercise rate, your body gets nearly all of this energy from burning body fat.

However, you can often burn glucose for energy if your body is fueled by carbohydrates. This makes burning and losing body fat much tricky for your body.

It is better to understand that although exercising can help you lose weight, it is necessary to get your diet correct first.

When the diet is correct, you can start tapping into its fat reserves for energy by using a well-designed ketogenic diet. This is what helps you to begin to burn and lose weight.

Once the body is used to the ketogenic diet, you can feel more vigorous. You would be best placed at that stage to change your menus to start building strength and muscles.

If you hit this point during your "normal ketogenic diet," you can change your diet to a "goal" or a "cyclical" ketogenic diet. These variations of the ketogenic diet allow you to use more carbohydrate for longer workouts.

Ketogenic Targeted Diet

The Targeted Ketogenic diet helps you to eat more carbohydrates during your workout. This diet helps you to exercise with high intensity while still in ketosis.

The carb intake in this window provides your muscles with the glucose required for your workouts effectively. The extra glucose can usually be used for around 30 minutes in this window and should not affect your entire metabolism.

The Ketogenic Targeted Diet is tailored for beginners or intermediate trainers. The TKD helps your carb intake to increase slightly. It does not, however, throw you out of ketosis and does not shock your system.

Ketogenic Cyclical Diet

For experienced athletes and bodybuilders, the Cyclical Ketogenic Diet is ideally adapted. It is commonly used for optimum performance in muscle building.

However, there is an unmistakable urge for most people to add some body fat. This is because the cyclical ketogenic diet (CKD) is easy to overeat.

The person follows the traditional ketogenic diet over 5 or 6 days in this variant of the ketogenic diet. It is then approved for 1 or 2 days to consume elevated carbohydrate quantities.

As a precaution, a novice will take nearly three weeks to return to ketosis entirely if he or she attempts the CKD. It takes real effort and advanced levels of practice to achieve a CKD successfully.

The Cyclical Ketogenic Diet aim is to eliminate ketosis temporarily. This window gives the body a chance to recharge the amount of glycogen in the muscles to undergo the next round of intensive training.

Therefore, the resulting glycogen build-up needs to be entirely removed during subsequent exercises to get back into ketosis. The strength of your preparation would also decide how many carbohydrates you eat.

Exercises in cardio

When you exercise at an intense pace, your body benefits immensely.

It helps to increase the quality of your heart and lung as you perform cardiovascular exercises. This also increases the rate at which the body absorbs energy and contributes to weight loss over time.

Cardio-exercise induces various physiological changes that have a beneficial effect on fat metabolism.

Cardiovascular activities help increase the oxygen supply by enhancing blood flow. In this way, body cells can oxidize and burn fat more efficiently.

It also increases the number of oxidative enzymes. The speed at which fatty acids are transported to the mitochondria for energy is thus substantially increased.

The sensitivity of muscles and fat cells to epinephrine is significantly improved during cardio-exercises. This raises the number of triglycerides released into the blood and the muscles used in energy intake.

Power exercise

Strong exercise tends to boost moods and also helps develop healthy bones. It also enables you to grow a good and balanced body overall.

Using a well-designed ketogenic, the muscles are maintained even during our strength training. Muscles are formed from muscle rather than fat or carbohydrates. Furthermore, since protein oxidation is less necessary in a ketogenic diet, strength training should not be an issue.

You have to question the bulky body to see results to get a more muscular body.

Training Interval

Interval training essentially alternates high-intensity and low-intensity training periods. You just have to: go quickly, go slowly, and repeat.

Although it sounds basic, interval training is one of the most effective ways to rapidly burn fat. In addition to burning fat during interval training, the 'after-burn effect' increases the metabolism for a more extended period of time.

Training Circuit: Aerobic + Power

Training on the circuit is simply the combination of aerobic activities and strength training. This mixture leads to overall fitness advantages.

This method of exercise blends aerobic exercises with resistance training without providing a time of rest between them. The absence of rest between the two exercises allows circuit training as successful as a high-intensity cardiovascular training exercise.

Yoga

The advantages of yoga are really its ability to help the body reduce stress hormone levels as well as improve insulin sensitivity.

Yoga lets you communicate with your body consciously. This will turn into a greater understanding of how your body functions and also improves your eating habits.

Chapter 2: Two Week Keto Diet Plan

Tips Before You Begin

If you just cook for yourself, freeze the remaining portions or chill them if appropriate, or half them.

Feel free to swap lunch for dinner, lunch brunch, and so on the same day. If you like, you can even switch the entire days.

Make the keto buns in advance (the whole recipe can be made with 10). Freeze the night before or in the oven before serving to hold fresh and defrost at room temperature.

You do not need snacks between foods, but if you do, make sure you have some keto-friendly snacks. Here's a list of snacks you can try, and a full list of diets is available here.

Deficient carbohydrate diets (less than 30 grams of net carbs) also have magnesium deficiencies. I recommend taking supplements with magnesium or adding high in magnesium snacks like nuts. Also, if you have any "keto-flu" signs, make sure you eat extra sodium.

This diet plan will not suit everyone-minor changes may be needed. Reduce portions of meat and eggs if you need less protein. Don't worry about a little protein waste, and it won't drive you out of ketosis. Protein actually retains appetite. If you want to less or add more fat, while making your changes, concentrate on added fatty and oils foods. Using Keto Diet Buddy to find your perfect macros!

Don't eat if you don't feel hungry, even if it means you're going to miss a meal.

Keto Diet Plan For First Weeks

Remember that no extra snacks are included in the nutrition facts of this meal plan. As individual needs vary, you can add healthy snacks to your appetite from this list. Simply add fat and protein-based foods or snacks if you feel hungry!

1st Day

Breakfast: Pudding chocolate

Total carbohydrates: 21.2 g, Net carbs: 6.3 g., Fiber: 14.9 g., Protein: 9.4 g., Calories: 329 kcal, Fat: 26,6 g., Magnesium: 63 mg.

Lunch : Easter Frittata

Total carbohydrates: 9.8 g. net carbs: 6.3 g., Fiber: 3.5 g., Protein: 25.5 g., calories: 503 kcal., fat: 37.5 g., magnesium: 40 mg.

Dinner: Hollandaise Sauce and Creamy Spinach with Salmon

Total carbohydrates: 6.5 g., net carbohydrate: 3.7 g, fiber: 2.8 g., Protein: 34 g., calories: 813 kcal., fat: 72.6 g., magnesium: 143 mg.

2nd Day:

Breakfast: Easter Frittata

Total carbs: 9.8 gr., net carbs: 6.3 g., fiber: 3.5 g, protein: 25.5 g., calorie: 503 kcal, fat: 37.5 g., magnesium: 40 mg.

Lunch: Salmon Stuffed Avocado

Total carbs: 13.9 g., net carbs (6.4 g); fiber: 7.5 g., proteins: 27 g.; calories: 463 kcal. fat: 34.6 g.; Calories: 75 mg.

Dinner: Simple Paprika Chicken with cauli-rice with 1 1/2 cup.

Total carbohydrates: 15 g, fiber: 5.3 g., calories: 714kcal, Protein: 27.2 g., net carbs: 9.8 g, Fat: 61.2 g., magnesium:65 mg.

3rd Day

Breakfast: All Day Keto Breakfast

Total carbohydrate agent (EMR): 15.5 g, fiber: 8.9 g., net carb: 6.6 g., Fat: 41.3 g., calories: 489 kcal, protein: 19.5 g., magnesium: 43 mg.

Lunch: Easter Frittata

Calorie: 503 kcal, power: 625 mg (31% EMR) magnesium: 40 mg (10% RDA), Total carbs: 9.8 g, fiber: 3.5 g, protein: 25.5 g, net carbs: 6.3 g, fat: 37.5 g,

Dinner: Easy Paprika Chicken with cauli-rice

Total carbs: 15 g., Net Carbs: 9.8 g., Fiber: 5.3 g., Protein: 27.2 g., Calories: 714 kcal., Fat: 51.2 g., Magnesium: 65 mg.

4th Day

Breakfast: Easter Frittata

Total carbs: 9.8 g, Net carbs: 6.3 g., Fiber: 3.5 g., Protein: 25.5 g., Calories: 515 kcal, Fat: 37.5 g., Magnesium: 30 mg.

Lunch: Easy Avocado and Egg Salad

Total carbohydrates: 13.7 g, Net Carbs: 6.1 g, Fiber: 7.6 g, Potassium: 17 g, Fat: 36.3 g, Magnesium: 60 mg (15% RDA), Calories: 436 kcal, Potassium: 875 mg (4% EMR).

Dinner: Paprika Chicken served with cauli-rice

Calorie: 714 kcal, potassium: 1018 mg (51% EMR) Total carbs: 15 g, fiber: 5.3 g, magnesium: 65 mg (16% RDA), net carb: 9.8 g, protein: 27.2 g., fat: 61.2 g.

5th Day

Breakfast: Chocolate Chia Pudding

Total carbohydrates: 21.2 g, Net carbs: 6.3 g., fiber: 14.9 g, Protein: 9.5 g., calories: 329 kcal, grade fat: 26.6 g., magnesium: 63 mg.

Lunch: Easy Paprika Chicken served with a cup of cauli-rice

Total carbs dioxide: 15 g, net carbs: 9.8 g, fiber: 5.3 g, proteins: 27.2 g., calories of 714 kcal, fat: 61.2 g., magnesium, 65 mg.

Dinner: Paleo Stuffed Avocado

Substitute the filling with if you don't like sardines:

3 oz / 85 g of salmon, 2 tbsp cream dill, cheese, lemon juice dash and salt

One spring onion, 1 tbsp mayo, lemon juice spring salt and dash, three oz/85 g tuna,

Overall carbohydrates: 19.5 g., net carbohydrates: 5.5 g, fiber: 14 g., Protein: 27.2 g, calorie: 633 g. k., fat: 52.6 g., magnesium: 99 mg.

6th Day

Breakfast: Pesto Scrambled Eggs

Magnesium: 26 mg (6 percent RDA), Calories: 467 kcal, potassium: 327 mg (16 percent EMR) Calories: 3.3 g, net carbs: 2.6 g, fiber: 0.7 g, protein: 20.4 g, fat: 41.5 g.

Lunch: Keto Bun with Avocado and Bacon Ultimate

1 Ultimate Keto Bun OR Nut-free Keto Buns, eaten with half and toasted:

- Two tbsp. of butter
- Two thin, crisped slices of bacon (30 g / 1.1 oz)
- Tomatoes 1/2 cup of cherry (75 g / 2,6 oz)
- Lettuce with two leaves (28 g / 1 oz).

Overall carbs dioxide: 24.1 g., Net carbs dioxide: 8 g., fiber: 16.2 g., fat: 61.5 g., calories: 673 kcal., protein: 17.4 g., magnesium: 131 mg.

Dinner: Salmon Stuffed Avocado

Calorie: 463 kcal, potassium: 1122 mg (EMR 56 million) Total carbs: 13,9 g, fiber: 7,5 g, net carbs: 6,4 g, magnesium: 75 mg (RDA 19%), protein: 27 g, fat: 34,6 g

7th Day

Breakfast: Hash Zucchini Breakfast

Overall carbs: 9.1 g, Net Carbs: 6.6 g, Fiber: 2.5 g, Protein: 17.4 g., Calorie: 422 kcal, Fat: 35.5 g., Magnesium: 53 mg.

Lunch: Keto Bun with Avocado & Bacon

1 Last Keto Bun OR Nut-free Buns, served in the form of:

- Two tbsp. of butter

- 2 green leaves (28 g / 1 oz)

- Two tiny bacon slices (30 g / 1.1 oz)

- 1/2 oz. (100 g) 1/2 oz.

- 1/2 cup of tomatoes with cherry (75 g / 2.6 oz)

Total carbs: 24,1 g., Fiber: 16,2 g., Net carb: 8 g., Protein: 17,4 g., Lip fat: 61,5 g., Calories: 673 kcal., Magnesium: 131 mg.

Dinner: Keto Gravy Great Pork Chops served with Creamy Keto Mash.

Total carbs: 16,3 g, 11,7 g net carbs, 4,7 gram fiber, 33 g protein, 702 kcal calories, 56,1 g fat, 1308 mg potassium (65% EMR) fiber 110 mg magnesium (28% RDA),

Keto Diet Plan for Second Weeks

1st Day

Breakfast: Smoothie Vanilla Keto

Total carbs: 5,6 g, Carbs net: 5,1 g, Fiber: 1,2 g, Potassium: 598 mg (30 per cent RDA), Calories: 566 kcal, Fat: 45,2 g, Magnesium: 26 mg.

Lunch: Simple Advocate and Egg Salad- Mayo rather than sour cream.

Fiber: 7.6 g., Total carbohydrate: 13.7 g, Net carbs: 6.1 g., Fat: 36.3 g., Kaloria: 436 kcal., Protein: 17 g., Magnesium: 60 mg.

Dinner: Keto Gravy Great Pork Chops with Creamy Keto Mash

Calories: 702 kcal, Net carbs: 11.7 g, Calories: 110 mg, Fat: 33 g, Magnesium: 110 mg (28% RDA), Fat: 56.1 g, Potassium: 1308 mg (65% EMR)

2nd Day

Breakfast: Pumpkin Pie Chia Pudding

Total carbs: 20.8 g., Net carbs: 6.6 g., Fiber: 14.2 g., Protein: 8.1 g., Calories: 295 kcal, Fat: 22.4 g., Magnesium: 39 mg.

Lunch: Avocado Stuffed Salmon

Calorie: 463 kcal, potassium: 1122 mg (56% EMR) magnesium: 75 mg (19% RDA), Total carbs: 13.9 g, fiber: 7.5 g, protein: 27 g, net carbs: 6.4 g, fats: 34.6 g, calories

Dinner: Great Ribeye Steak served with Creamy Keto Mash with Gremolata

Total carbohydrate: 12.7 g, net carbohydrate: 8.3 g, fiber: 4.4 g, protein: 41.7 g, fat: 90.1 g, magnesium: 97 mg, calories: 1024 kcal, potassium: 1477 mg.

3rd day

Breakfast: Eggs Scrambled Pesto

Total carbohydrates: 3,3 g., net carbohydrates: 2,6 g., fiber: 0,7 g, protein: 20,4 g., calories:467 kcal., fat: 41,5 g., magnesium: 25 mg., potassium: 327 mg.

Lunch: Modern salad Tricolore

Overall carbs: 17.6 g., Net carbs: 8.6 g., Fiber: 9 g., Potassium: 19.2 g., Calories: 581 kcal., Fat: 50.7 g., Magnesium: 70 mg.

Dinner:Creamy Keto Mash pan-roasted salmon

One medium salmon fillet (150g/5.3 oz) fried on 1 tbsp ghee, herbs like dill, seasoned with salt and pepper, and a splash of citrus juice.

1 Creamy Keto Mash Serving

Total carbohydrate content: 11.7 g, net carbs: 7.8 g, fiber: 3.9 g, protein: 36.1 g, calories: 660 kcal, magnesium: 79 mg, fat: 51.9 g, potassium: 1253 mg (63% EMR).

4th Day

Breakfast: Keto Smoothie chocolate

Calories: 570 kcal, potassium: 560 mg. (28% EMR) magnesium: 45 mg (11% RDA), Gross carbs: 6.2 g., fiber: 2.8 g, protein: 34.5 g, fat: 46 g.

Lunch: Simple Avocado and Egg Salad-mayo instead of sour cream

Total carbs dioxide: 13.7 g, Net carbs: 6.1 g, Fiber: 7.6 g, Calories: 436 kcal, Protein: 17 g, Fat: 36.3 g, Magnesium: 60 mg (15 percent RDA).

Dinner

Serve with buttered Brussels sperm sprigs and with keto sauce optionally (cheese sauce is not in the nutritional facts, + 200 kcal and net carbs 1 g) Spicy Chorizon meatballs.

Total carbohydrates: 17,6 g, 6,6 g, Protein: 31,8 g, Net carbs: 11 g, Fat: 49,5 g, Magnesium: 92 mg (23% RDA), Calories: 627 kcal,

5th Day

Breakfast: Eggs Pesto Scrambled

Calories: 467 kcal, magnesium: 25 mg (6 percent RDA), net carbs: 2.6 g, potassium: 327 mg (16 percent EMR): 4.3 g, fiber: 0.7 g, fat: 41.5 g protein: 20.4 g,

Lunch: Modern Salad Tricolore

Total carbs: 17,6 g, 9 g, Net carbs: 19,2 g, 8,6 g, 50,7 gr. fat, 581 kcal, 70 mg (19 percent RDA), 942 mg (47 percent EMR) magnesium.

Dinner

Serve with Buttered Brussels Sprouts with Keto Cheese (cheese sauce is not in nutritional details included, + net carbs 1 g with 200 kcal)

Total carbohydrate: 17.6 g., Carbohydrate net: 11 g., fiber 6.6 g., Protein: 31.8 g., Calories: 627 kcal, Gas fat: 49.5 g., Magnesium: 92 mg.

6th Day

Breakfast: Hash Zucchini Breakfast

Total carbs: 9.1 g, Net carbs: 6.6 g, Fiber: 2.5 g, Protein: 17.4 g, Calories: 422 kcal, Fat: 35.5 g, Magnesium: 53 mg (13% RDA)

Lunch: Good salad mackerel

Total carbs: 16,1 g, net carbs: 7,6 g., fiber: 8,5 g., protein: 27,3 g., calories: 609 kcal., fat: 49,9 g., magnesium: 133 mg.

Dinner

Serve with buttered Brussels spicy chorizo meatballs and optionally Keto sauce (cheese sauce is not in information on nutritious food + 1 g of net carbs with 200 kcal)

Total carbohydrates: 17.6 g., net carbohydrates: 11 g., Protein: 31.8 g., calories: 627 kcal., fat: 49.5 g., magnesium: 92 kg. (23% RDA).

7th day

Breakfast: Keto Breakfast All Day

Overall carbs: 15.5 g, proteins: 19.5 g.; fiber: 8.7 g, calories: 489 kcal; net carbs: 6.6 g; fat: 41.3 g.; magnesium: 43 mg.

Lunch: Avocado Stuffed Salmon

Total carbs: 13.8 g., Net carbs: 6.5 g., Fiber: 7.5 g., Protein: 27 g., Calories: 463 kcal., Fat: 34.6 g., Magnesium: 75 mg.

Dinner

Spicy chorizo meatballs, with buttered Brussels springs and optionally with Cheese Sauce (The Cheese sauce is not in fact included, + 1 gram of carbohydrate and 200 kcal)

Fat: 6,6 g 17,6 g, Fiber, 11 g net carbohydrates, 31.8 g protein, 49,5 g fat, 627kcal calories, 92 mg magnesium (23% RDA), 1029 mg potassium (52% EMR)

Recipe Substitutions

You can try here alternatives if you don't like certain ingredients or if you are intolerant to certain foods.

- Try any of the paleo-friendly diets in this list if you're dairy intolerant. And for those who don't consume meat, there is a keto-friendly vegetarian diet.
- Pork, lamb and fatty (mackerel, salmon, and sardines) can be replaced because their diet profile is close
- Use the beef chorizo or roast beef instead if you don't eat bacon.
- You should try Nut-free Keto Buns instead of Keto Buns Ultimate
- Chia Pudding – all three recipes mentioned on the schedule (pumpkin, berry and chocolate) do not have to be prepared.

Everyone has similar food facts that can be used interchangeably.

- Chocolate Keto Smoothie and Pumpkin Smoothie can be supplemented by the following recipes

The use of these alternatives would not modify the reality of nutrition substantially. Please be aware that the shopping list is created with the regular alternative.

Good Low-Carb Snacks And Supplements

- 1 piece of FAT BOMBS
- Almond milk, Cream coffee or Cappuccino Low Carb
- 1 cup of bone bud
- 1/2 pink Himalayan salt avocado
- 1 hard-boiled egg with pink Himalayan salt (you're still in the refrigerator)
- Crispy slices of bacon (prepare and refrigerate)
- Roll-up ham and cheese
- 2-3 celery sticks of 2 tbsp. Home-made cocoon and pecan butter or any nut butter.
- Fermented foodstuffs: kimchi, sauerkraut (add to breakfast), small quantities of kombucha (carbs)
- Pork rinds or chicken crackles rather than chips (avoid additive products
- Nuts and sown seed, handful, raw or roasted with marine salt (net carbs per 1 oz): pecans -1.2 g, almonds-2.7 g, walnuts-2 g, hazelnuts-2 g, macadamias-1.5 g, nuts-1.4 g, pine sown-3.2 g, pine nuts-2.7 g, pumpkin seed-1.3 g)-nuts are advisable to soak.
- Berry blackberries (net of carbs per serving: one-half cup of blackberries-3,1 g, one/2 cup of raspberries-3,3 g, one-half cup of strawberries-4,1 g or one-quarter of a cup of blueberries-4,5 g).
- Cocoa oil (for a tablespoon of cocoon oil in silicone ice trays, keep in the refrigerator for a fast fat-burning snack)

Low-Carb and Keto Diet Fast Food Menu Choices

For those that eat low-carbs or keto diets, in every fast-food place or restaurant, you will almost always eat something. Plan ahead.. Check their menu and nutrition details online at home or using your mobile before visiting a restaurant. Before being tempted by menu items you cannot have on a low-carb diet, you still have to know the healthier choices.

Here are several restaurants and those things that I considered to be the lowest (and most emotionally satisfying) choices in order to make it easier to find the quickest keto-friendly alternative. These are not all ideal choices, but if you have no other choices due to restrictions on time or on the venue, they would be in a pinch.

It is a tremendous aid for fast-food places to post nutritional content. Every day it is easier to obey the keto diet. The number of carbs I have mentioned is estimated and is NET grams.

Usually, there is a salad option wherever you are. Remove the bun at the Burger joints, and instead, several places sell salad wraps. Chicken is not expected to have breading.

It helps to have a handy knife and fork in your car or wallet. Big, pieces of salad are on your table in small juicy burgers, or in your lap. Tiny, flimsy plastic foods also make it hard to eat. Take out and enjoy your own robust utensils!

There are already some unambiguous general guidelines for food choices:

- Miss the wrap or bun
- Miss pasta, rice or potato
- Salads-no croutons. Caesar, Ranch, Blue Cheese, Chipotle with low sugar dressing options. Look at the name that will tell you, stuff like "honey" in the sweet dressing Dijon or "sweet" – generally, it's not the right choice. Check the ingredient for carbohydrates that are higher.
- Chicken-Pick grilled or sprinkled. Keep away from any breaded chicken.

McDonalds-go for any chicken (2 g) or burger (zero-g) without the bun, with cheese, mustard, mayo, onion and so on. No ketchup. Attach side lettuce (3 g). The Caesar's salad with grilled chicken or the grilled chicken's bacon ranch salad is 9 g.

Burger king: burger (zero-g) without the bun and topped with ointments, mayo, cheese, mustard, etc. No ketchup. The chicken sandwich is 3 g without the bun. BEWARE – you might think that the burger is tiny, but 19 g of carbs, so that's a whole day of keto carbs. Attach side lettuce (3 g). The garden salad is 8 g tender grill with no dressing or croutons. The chicken salad is not an option. Do not try.

Freshly fried apple and 5 g net carbs WITHOUT caramels are not fried.

Subway-Subway can probably miss if you can. The wraps and buns are rich in carbohydrates. I suppose you might have them in a wrapper sans bun, but it doesn't sound enticing. I don't have any details on the carb count for any bunless sub, but you can probably figure it out – chicken or pepperoni is all right, but is "Sweet onion" chicken, all right? No idea. No idea. Stick to the salads, but remember that you're just going to get iceberg (4 g).

Carl's Junior and Hardees — this chain provides a "lettuce wrap"— your burger wrapped in a large piece of salad for quick low-carb food. I choose to bring my own fork instead. Bun less choices without croutons, grilled chicken salad is 10 g. The salad on the side is 3 g.

Wendy's-Again, in a lettuce wrap or package, you can carry your burger. Any topping burger. Mayo's got maize syrup and is 1 g. The fillet of the chicken grill is 1 g. You can order it in the sandwich of a chicken club or the ultimate grill sandwich. Best salads: chicken Caesar (7 g), blue grilled chicken salad. Side salads for Caesar 6 g or 2 g.

Pizza Hut and other pizza Locations-Pizza without crust can be consumed. You need to eat two times as much, but if you can't resist a group or a dinner in a pizza, slice the cheesy tops off and eat the tremendous messy pile of cheese and toppings. A side salad is a good extra. Otherwise, simply choose to make pizza with low carbs crust at home.

Mongolian Grill-YES! Load your bowl with chicken, shrimp, onion and mushrooms, then add a sauce of Asian black bean. I know that beans have carbs, but the sauce label says 1 gram of carbs per ounce (every sauce is clearly marked). Add some garlic and wait before the griller does its job. Of course, you miss the heat, the tortillas and the rice. Ask the waiting workers not to carry them to the table.

Italian restaurants-They requires a bit of cleverness, but they can be fancy! Ideas: how about the Italian chicken Marsala? Make sure the pasta doesn't come. Replace broccoli or some other keto-friendly lateral dish or a large salad. Chicken picante is also a chance.

Restaurants in Mexico and China are the toughest since any low-carb choices are not the primary reason to go to the restaurant. I like to get a big burrito with at a Mexican restaurant and spread out the soft tortilla like a plate. Eat the ingredients and throw the tortilla.

Wings Anywhere-Basic buffalo sauce is typically OK, as is Parmesan garlic.

Comfort shops can also be the right choice! 7-11 has hard-boiled packs of eggs, slim jims, cheese slabs, almonds and rinds of pork. Pork rinds come with the taste of a barbecue, and they are ZERO carbs.

Remember to keep bread, potatoes, pasta, rice, fries and tortilla at bay. And watch for maize starch, bread crumbs and other fillers. You will be able to find balanced keto and low-carb choices while dining and stick to your good keto diet plan with the right schedule and attitude.

Anyone who wants to lose weight is safe with the ketogenic diet.

Differences Between Total Carbs vs Net Carbs

As soon as you start exploring the keto diet, you discover that you have to considerably limit your carbohydrate intake to follow it successfully. But how much? What? Some reports say that your consumption should be restricted to 20 total carbs a day, while others say twenty net carbs a day. What is the difference between gross carbs dioxide and net carbs dioxide? Everything you need to know will be clarified here so that you can determine the regular intake of carb which is right for you.

What is the purpose of limiting carbohydrates?

To know why you need to understand about the net and total carbs, it is a good idea to understand the role of carbs limitation in the keto diet:

The whole purpose of a ketogenic diet is to keep your body in a ketosis state. This is why the body based upon energy fat rather than the carbohydrates (sugar), and if you measure it, ketone levels are at least 0,5 mol / L.

Ketosis is only accomplished by significantly reducing your carb intake long enough to train your body to generate ketones at stored and ingested fats the use them as energy. If you are in ketosis, the goal is to remain and maximize its many advantages. The only way to do that is to keep your carb intake minimal.

But just how much?

How many carbs do you need to eat on a keto diet every day?

Fortunately, it is not arbitrary to eat the sum of carbs on a keto diet. Actually, it is empirical, although the complexities that we describe here create some confusion:

Comprehensive carbs

It is generally appropriate for doctors to restrict their consumption of carb to 20 grams of total carbs a day in people adopting a ketogenic diet for medically medicinal purposes including cancer or epilepsy. Strict adherence ensures that higher cetone levels optimize the benefits.

In this case, 'complete carbs' sounds like the entire amount of carbs eaten within one day. It is crucial to monitor the consumption of your foods with a tracker, which is often called macros since carbs can sneak in your diet easily.

Carbs Net

Experts believe that almost everyone will remain firmly in ketosis (that is, hold ketone levels at least 0.5 mol / L or more) if they eat 20 grams of net carbs a day.

This is where keto beginners could be mistaken: "Net carbs" are not the same as "absolute carbohydrates."

Net carbs are the total grams of every food except the grams of fiber and sucrose alcohol. (Alcohols in sugar and fiber are subtracted when the body is not digested.)

Here's the underlying formula:

A portion of fiber and sugar alcohols can be subtracted from total carbs to calculate net carbs.

Formula: total carbs minus fiber (or half of IMO) minus half the carbs from sugar alcohols (other than erythritol) = net carbs.

This is an example of a measurement of net carb, using 1 cup of cauliflower rice:

One cup cauliflower rice contains 4.8 g of total carbohydrates and 3.2 g of fiber. To obtain the net carbs, you extract the fiber (3.2 grams) of the total carbs (4.8 grams), leaving you with 1.6 grams of net carbs (i.e., 3.2 grams of carbs = 1.6 Grams of net carbs for one cup of cauliflower).

If you adopt a keto diet due to weight loss or general health purposes, you have to remain under 20 net carbs a day. It is simpler to do, helps you to consume much more vegetables and other nutritious foods with carbs and, as we have said, also permits ketosis.

Let us now pursue an example of food containing sugar alcohol. There are several ketos and low-carb products that use sugar-based alcohol-based sweeteners in order to sweeten foodstuffs without adding carbohydrates (or adding limited carbohydrates in the case of such sugar alcohol). However, there are also recipes for sugar alcohol. We suggest erythritol sweetener. It contains no carbs at all and does not affect blood sugar levels, unlike other sugar alcohols. So, we will use home-made keto whipped cream for this example (two cup of high whipping cream and two erythritol teaspoons, whipped together).

In this case, a whipped cream contains 32 grams of carbohydrates and 0 dietary fiber (or 32 whole carbohydrates), while erythritol includes 8 grams of total carbohydrate and 8 grams of fiber.

Your carb edge or sustainable individuality checking

After three or more months of substantial ketosis, some people want to test their "carb edge," to decide if they can eat more than 20 net carbs a day while staying in ketosis. You can do this by gradually increasing your daily intake of carbohydrates and monitoring your glucose and ketones every day for glucose spikes or ketoses.

Testing yourself for bio-individuality or how your unique body reacts to certain foods is also common. For instance, some people have a glucose spike with some sugar alcohols or milk. Checking the glucose and ketones before and after ingestion of dubious foods helps you to find out if a diet susceptibility impedes the ability to remain in ketosis and thrive.

Total carbs are the sum of all your carbs in a day. Net carbs are measured by taking total fiber and sugar alcohols. What is best for you to adopt a ketogenic diet depends on your objectives. If you adopt a ketogenic diet for medical purposes, it is easier to start with 20 TOTAL carbs a day. It is the best idea to test your ketones when seeking your carb edge and see if food sensitivities impact your performance. It is also important to verify before you start a diet with your primary health care provider.

Chapter 3: Keto Dieting: Foods You Should Have in Kitchen

A ketogenic diet uses high fat and low carbohydrate to burn fat rather than glucose. Many people know the Atkins diet, but the keto method further limits carbohydrates.

When we are in a place where fast food and processed food, avoiding carbohydrates can be a challenge, but careful preparation can aid.

Prep meals and snacks at least a week in advance, so you're not just caught with high carbohydrates. Check for online recipes; there are a few nice recipes to choose from. Take a look at the keto diet, search and stick to your favorite recipes.

Some products are staples of a keto diet. Make sure that these things are available:

1. Eggs-Used in quiche, omelets, low carb pizza, hard fried as snack, and more; you have the significant chance of succeeding in eggs, if you want eggs, on this diet.

2. Bacon- Do I need justification? Breakfast, burger topper, salad garnish, try a bowl of BLT tossed in mayo

3. Cream cheese-hundreds of the recipe, crusts of pizza, main dishes, desserts

4. Shredded cheese-Scatter with taco meat in a tub, microwave chips, salad tops, low-carbs pizza and enchiladas

5. Dark greens and spinach – Load up on green veggies; have enough to get a quick salad when hunger hits

6. EZ-Sweetz Sweetener- Just use a few drops instead of sugar and is the natural and easy-to-use artificial sweetener

7. Cauliflower-This low-carb veggie is fresh or frozen by itself, tossed into olive oil and fried, mashed into counterfeited potatoes, chopped or shredded and used in place of rice under main dishes, in low carbs and keto pizzas, etc.

8. Ground beef-Make a massive burger and top all kinds of cheese, saute mushrooms, grilled onions. or crumble and cook in provolone taco cookery; throw in the dish a tortilla salad of lettuce, avocado, cheese, sour cream

9. Almonds are a great and nutritious snack (flat or flavoured), but be sure to count them while you eat, because carbs can add. Habanero, chocolate, salt and vinegar and other flavors are included.

The Keto diet is a flexible and fascinating way to lose weight and provides several delicious food options. Keep the ten items in your fridge, freezer and larder, and you can put some delightful keto meals and snacks together at a time.

Anybody who wants to lose weight has a ketogenic diet. Visit the Safe Keto website, a helpful resource for keto dieters to provide access to food and dietary information.

Why Is Keto Diet So Effective For People +50

Keto has become a popular diet in recent years and a food plan preferred by people of all ages. Having said that, this dietary roadmap could bring particularly significant health benefits to people over 50 years of age.

The decreased consumption of carbohydrates is said to gradually position the bodies of participating dieters through a biological and metabolic phase known as ketosis.

Once ketosis has been established, medical researchers believe the body is particularly useful in burning fat and converting it into energy. In addition, the organism is expected to metabolize fat in chemicals that are classified as ketones and also provide essential sources of energy during this process.

An accelerator of this is an intermittent fasting process where the restricting of carbohydrates allows the body to enter the next available energy source or ketones that are extracted from stored fat.

There are a variety of other unique keto diets, including:

(TKD) Targeted

Many who engage in this edition add small quantities of carbohydrates to their diets increasingly.

(CKD) Cyclical

Members of this food plan use cyclically like every few days or weeks carbohydrates.

High-Protein

As part of their eating plans, high-protein observers consume more massive amounts of protein.

SKD (Standard)

This more widely used version of diet generally dramatically reduces carbohydrate concentrations (perhaps less than 5 per cent), protein-laden and a high volume of fatty products (in some instances up to 75 per cent of all dietary requirements).

In some instances, in standard or high-protein variants the regular dietitian or anyone new to the keto diet participates. Cyclical and targeted modifications are typically created by professional athletes or individuals with exceptional dietary needs.

Foods Suggested

Keto dietary adherents are advised to eat foods like meat products, fatty fish, milk, cream and butter, eggs, salts, low carbohydrate-level products, pepper and many other spices, various seeds and nuts, and oils such as coconut and olive. Some foods, on the other hand, should be avoided or strictly limited. These include beans and legumes, numerous fruits, alcohol, high-sugar food, and grain products.

Keto diet advantages for people over 50 years old

Keto diet participants, especially those 50 years of age or older, are said to have several potential health benefits, including:

Increased Mental and Physical Resources

As people get older, energy levels can fall for a number of environmental and biological reasons. Keto diet followers also experience an increase in strength and vitality. One explanation that occurs is because the body burns excess fat, which in turn becomes electricity. In addition, systemic ketone synthesis appears to increase brain capacity and stimulate cognitive functions such as attention and memory.

Enhanced sleep

People appear to sleep less as they grow older. Keto dieters often gain more from workouts and become more tired. This can lead to more extended and more fruitful rest periods.

Staff wear

Aging people also experience a higher metabolism than their younger days. Long-term dieters have more increased blood sugar regulation, which can improve their metabolic rate.

Loss of weight

Faster and more effective metabolism of fat helps the body lose stored fat, which can prevent extra pounds from being thrown away. Adherents are also thought to have a decreased appetite, which might result in reduced caloric intake.

Holding weight off is particularly important as an adult as they may need fewer calories a day compared to 20s or even 30s as living there. However, it is still essential for older adults to get nutrient-rich food from this diet.

Because it is common for aging adults to lose muscle and strength, a nutritionist may prescribe a high-protein specific ketogenic diet.

Protection from specific diseases

Keto dieters over age 50 will minimize their risk of developing illnesses such as diabetes, psychiatric disorders such as Alzheimer's, different cardiovascular conditions, other forms of cancer, Parkinson's disease.

Aging

Some consider aging to be the key risk factor for human disorders. The reduction of aging is, therefore, the logical step to decrease these disease risk factors.

Good news from the technical explanation of the earlier ketosis process shows the increased energy of the young as a consequence, and the use of fat as a source of fuel means the body will go through the process of misinterpretation of signs to suppress the mTOR signal and to make it clear that a lack of glucose may lead to slowing aging.

In general, several studies have shown that caloric limitations can help delay aging and even increase lifespan for years. With the ketogenic diet, it is possible to have an effect on anti-aging without reducing calories. Vascular aging can also be influenced by an intermittent fasting process with the keto diet.

When anyone fasts intermittently or on a keto diet, it is presumed that the BHB or Beta-Hydroxybutyrate causes anti-aging results.

To be sure, more than researching this diet, advantages, positive effects and side effects are required, particularly for older adults on the internet and in newspapers. Specifically, her or his medical professional should be consulted on specific issues.

Simple Tips and Exercise To Lose Weight

There are different ways to quickly lose weight and melt the fat immediately. However, most of them are disappointed when you know that weight loss shortcuts do not last long. Weight loss is a mixture of a well-formulated diet and a vigorous routine. If you wonder how to lose weight, here are a few easy tips for weight loss and exercises to minimize weight and weight-loss.

1. Train your mind.

Weight loss requires a healthy diet, intense exercise but above all emotional belief. Before beginning a weight loss journey, mentally remember why you are taking this step and hold this justification for keeping you going and stopping you from eating comfort food.

2. Stop foods that are high in sugar.

Insulin is our body's fat-storage hormone, and sucrose foods like desserts release insulin. This immediately increases our blood sugar level, which in turn contributes to fat accumulation. Downward insulin also acts as a detox for the body that helps the kidneys to eliminate extra sodium or nitrates that can cause bloating. It is critical that fizzy drinks that also cause gas are absolutely cut out.

3. Don't leave a food group out.

The weight loss industry renders one food group or the other the worst for the body every year. It is best to include all fats, proteins and carbohydrates in our diet. Protein-rich food has proven to improve metabolism and minimize cravings.

4. Your savior is watered.

Make sure you stay hydrated all day long with water and other fluids. At least eight glasses of water must be drunk a day to avoid this bloating. I suggest a glass of water with lemon right after you wake up.

5. Fiber is necessary for a safe intestine.

Foods such as vegetables are high in fiber, avoiding constipation and helping you get a flat belly fast. It also helps to enhance the metabolism and immune system in the long term.

6. Keep away from fad diets.

Today's market is filled with diets like the GM diet, Atkins, Keto diet, which have a significant long-term effect on bodies. Try to be careful and eat everything but moderately.

Diet strategy for a loss of weight:

Here is a regular diet you can use for weight loss, please consult your nutritionist before following any diet. Everyone's body is unique; not everyone can use a sole diet.

Breakfast: 3 egg whites OR Oatmeal with green tea and fruit.

Mid-morning snack: 150 gms of vinegar/soya chicken OR 1 steamed 6-inch maize tortilla with fresh or grilled vegetables (for example onions, peppers and tomatoes) and no-added salt salsa.

Lunch: grilled fish, 1 cup of other vegetables, broccoli OR 2 cups of mixed greens, sliced, dressed in balsamic vinegar aged

Half afternoon snack: chickpeas salad OR banana and an apple.

Dinner: Shake the protein with any protein (chicken, tofu, fish.)

Exercise schedule for weight loss

Will you need a weight loss workout? Join a workout routine to do a new thing every day. Engage in high cardiovascular exercises such as dancing, Zumba, jumping, but also the gym. It is necessary to retain muscle mass, and even after the workout, it burns fat. A fast HIIT (High-Intensity Interval Training) exercise is a perfect way to absorb a healthy 1000 calories.

If you obey the above points, you will lose weight healthily! The trick is always a diet along with some exercise.

Fat Loss Diet Ultimate

The diet of the keto. What's the diet for the keto? It's literally when you get your body to use your BODYFAT as the main source of energy rather than carbohydrates. The keto diet is a common way to quickly and effectively lose weight.

The Science Secret

You have to consume high-fat diets and low protein with or barely any carbs in order to bring the body into a ketogenic state. The ratio should be roughly 80% fat and 20% protein. This is the first two days' guideline. If you have ketogenic intake and lower fat, then the ratio will be about 65% fat, 30 % protein and 5% carbohydrates. To spare muscle tissue, protein is increased. If the body eats carbohydrates, it triggers an insulin spike, meaning that the pancreas free insulin (helps retain amino acids glycogen, and too much fatty calories as well) so good sense tells us that if we remove carbs the insulin won't store excess calories as fat.

Now your body does not have any carbs as an energy source that your body wants to find. This works really well if you're going to lose fat on your body. The body breaks down body fat and uses it instead of carbohydrates as energy. This condition is referred to as ketosis. This is the state in which you want your body to be; it makes complete sense to lose your weight while holding your muscles.

Now about the diet and how to prepare it. You need to take AT LEAST a gram of protein per pound of LEAN MASS. That's what improves muscle tissue regeneration and repair after exercise and so on. Recall the ratio? Sixty-five per cent fat and 30 % protein. Ok, if you weigh 150 lbs,that is 150 g of protein a day, the X4, which is 600 calories (amount of calories per gram of protein). You should get the rest of your calories from fat. If your calorie maintenance amounts to 3000, you have to eat around 500 less, which means that about 1900 calories would come from fats if you need 2500 calories daily! You need to consume fats to fuel your body, and burn off the body fat in exchange! You have to eat fats that is the law of this diet! The value of eating dietary fats and keto is that you're not going to feel hungry. Fat digestion is sluggish, which allows you to feel 'please.'

You're going to do it Monday-Friday and then "carb-up" on the weekend. After your last training on Friday, the carbs begins. You have to take a liquid carbohydrate and your whey shake after exercise. This helps generate an insulin spike which helps to urgently remedy, which replenish the nutrients your body needs in muscle stores. Eat what you want throughout this point (carb up), crisps, pasta, ice cream or/and pizzas. This will be good for you, as it will refill you and restore your body's nutritional needs in the coming week. On Sunday, the no high fat, moderate protein diet begins. The best cure is to keep your body in ketosis and to burn fat as energy.

Another advantage of ketosis is that when you reach the state of ketosis and burn the fat, you are filled with carbohydrates. After you have loaded carbs, you'll look as complete as ever (with less body fat!), great for the weekends when you go to the beach or a party!

Now let the diet rundown.

- -Must reach the ketosis state by removing carbohydrates from the diet when taking moderate / low high fat protein.
- -You have to take some sort of fiber to keep your pipes as open as ever when you know what I mean.
- -At least one gram of protein per pound of lean mass must be included in ketosis protein consumption.
- -That's a lot of it! It takes no effort to consume carbs the entire week as many foods have carbohydrates but note that you are

greatly rewarded for your dedication. You should not end up in ketosis for weeks because it is dangerous, and you will end up using protein as a fuel source which is a no go.

Mixing MCT Oil with Ketogenic Diet Plan

We still talk about must-haves in life. If you drive a high-end vehicle, you have to drive motor oil through the top of the rows. If you race on a high track level, state-of-the-art running shoes are a must. When you celebrate a big quarter at the workplace, you have to have the finest whiskey. I would recommend to you that if you take a ketogenic lifestyle seriously, MCT Oil is a must-have.

MCT Oil delivers a healthy dose of the very fuels that make the body a fat-burning machine and holds it. Contrary to LCTs, MCTs skip most of the digestion mechanism through which other fats pass. MCTs, behave more like a carbohydrate in how they are directly sent to the liver where they are used for energy.

MCT makes complete sense for your ketogenic diet for several reasons, but we have some of the significant benefits of MCT Oil in your Ketogenic diet plan to help you understand how they can play a crucial role in your nutrition.

As you already know, MCTs go to the liver and behave "carb-like," so that LCTs cannot. In theory, you can initiate ketosis by following the following steps:

1. No Breakfast.

If you are not using Keto for a long time and want to return to a fat-burning state quickly, a combination of MCT oil and fasting will do the job. Eat a low carb meal, or even save meal, and wake up and eat no breakfast! Drink a cup of coffee instead and put in your coffee a tablespoon or two of MCT oils and head out.

2. Replacement of meals with MCT Oil

Another advantage is the use of MCT Oil as a meal substitute for your Ketogenic Diet strategy.

This quite looks like the previous fasting point with MCT Oil but, aside from your substitution by some MCT Oil, you are still consuming some daily ketogenic meals.

MCT Oil's capacity to satisfy your appetite is one of the advantages. As long as it sounds scary initially to rely only on a few tablespoons of oil to replace meals, your body will become more and more accustomed. MCTs will substitute what is usually there and decrease the fierce badger and hunger cravings.

3. Ramp your Ketogenic MCT dishes

The flexibility of MCT Oil is incredible. Let's assume that you're in Ketosis already, but you're able to eat a salad for your regular carbs, and you want to keep it on Keto life for 100. This is easy! It is easy! Using MCT as the basis for your dressing, and you'll always be burning fat after your greens have been down!

And what if you don't bake? What if you want to do a jog and introduce MCT Oil's energy efficiency? How about a good sports drink from Keto?! All you need is water, and then squeeze in some lemon juice, and for long sun workouts, you'll have a better non-sugary sports drink.

There are some ways to skin the cat, and there are many ways to improve your Ketogenic Diet. MCTs are necessary for your body to become the fat-burning machine. Unfortunately, you won't always be able to get the right amount alone from your diet, you will need to improve it, and MCT Oil is that improve.

Life is packed with "must-have," and your diet doesn't slip out of the mantra realm. If you want to live a genuinely ketogenic lifestyle, you'll invest in and incorporate the right fuels as effectively as possible. And what is the advantage of MCT in the Ketogenic Diet plan? Response: performance. A healthy diet that allows you more time to do what you enjoy and fosters a productive lifestyle.

At Keys to Ketosis, we work to create, inform and empower the Ketogenic Community! If you have ever wanted ketosis or are searching for ways to change your ketogenic lifestyle.

Chapter 4: Benefits and Uses of Keto Diet

Your body becomes more a fat burner than a carbohydrate-dependent machine when it has a ketogenic diet. Several research studies have linked increased carbohydrate intake to several disorders, including diabetes and insulin resistance.

Carbohydrates are generally easily absorbable and can therefore be easily stored in the body as well. Carbohydrate digestion starts right from the moment you put it in your mouth.

As soon as you start to chew them, amylase (the enzymes digesting carbohydrate) in your saliva already acts on the food that contains carbohydrates.

Carbohydrates are further broken down in the stomach. They are absorbed into the bloodstream as they reach the small intestines. Carbohydrates naturally increase blood sugar levels as they enter the bloodstream.

This rise in blood sugar promotes immediate blood circulation of insulin. The higher the increase in blood sugar, the more insulin is produced.

Insulin is a hormone that eliminates excess sugar from the bloodstream to reduce blood sugar. The sugar and carbohydrate you consume are taken by insulin and processed in muscle tissues as glycogen and in adipose tissue as fat for potential energy usage.

However, when the body is exposed continuously to such high levels of blood glucose, what is known as insulin resistance will develop. This can cause obesity easily because the body stores excess glucose quickly. This disorder may also result in health problems such as cardiovascular and diabetes diseases.

Keto diets high in fat and low in carbohydrates, along with many health problems minimized and strengthened.

One of the essential things a ketogenic diet can do is balance the insulin levels and restore leptin signals. Reduced levels of insulin in the bloodstream make you feel more total and less craves for a more extended period of time.

Ketogenic diets medical benefits

The ketogenic diet has been applied and incorporated considerably. Keto diets are also indicated in a variety of medical conditions as part of the treatment plan.

Epilepsy

This is essentially the critical explanation of why the ketogenic diet has evolved. The incidence of epileptic seizures for some cause is decreased when patients are treated with a keto diet.

Pediatric forms of epilepsy are the most vulnerable to the keto diet. Some children have seizure removal after a couple of years of utilizing a keto diet.

Children with epilepsy usually are supposed to rapidly start their ketogenic diets for a few days.

Cancer

Research indicates that, when paired with some medications and procedures, ketogenic diets can increase their therapeutic effectiveness against tumor growth under a "press-pulse" model.

It is also encouraging to remember that ketogenic diets contribute to the remission of cancer cells.

Disease of Alzheimer

There are many signs that the memory functions of Alzheimer's patients improve after a ketogenic diet has been employed.

Ketones are a great source of alternative energy for the brain, especially when it is insulin resistant. Ketones can provide substrates (cholesterol) for neurons and membranes that are weakened to repair. All this helps to enhance patients with Alzheimer's memory and cognition.

Diabetics

Carbohydrates are widely accepted as the primary cause of diabetes. There are greater chances of optimizing blood sugar regulation by growing the consumed glucose by using a ketogenic diet.

In addition, it will significantly increase its overall efficacy if a keto diet is paired with other diabetes treatment plans.

Gluten Allergy

Many people with gluten allergy haven't even been diagnosed. However, there was a change in associated symptoms such as digestive pain and bloating following a ketogenic diet.

The majority of foods rich in carbohydrates are high in gluten. Thus, the use of a keto diet eliminates a lot of gluten intake to a minimum by eliminating a wide range of carbohydrates.

Loss of weight

This is probably the most popular "intentional" use of today's ketogenic diet. It found a niche in the mainstream dietary pattern for itself. Keto diets have been part of many diets because of its well-known side effect of helping to lose weight.

While many initially maligned, the number of favorable outcomes in weight loss has enabled the ketogenic to better be accepted as an effective weight loss program.

In addition to the aforementioned medical advantages, ketogenic diets often provide some general health benefits, including the following.

Improved sensitivity to insulin

Obviously, this is the first goal of a ketogenic diet. It helps to regulate insulin levels, boosting fat intake.

Preservation of muscle

Protein is oxidized and helps sustain magnetic muscle. Losing lean muscle mass slows down a person's metabolism as the muscles are usually highly metabolic. Using a keto diet helps to build your muscles while your body burns fat.

PH and respiratory function regulated.

A keto diet helps lower lactate and increases both pH and respiratory function. A ketosis disorder thus helps to keep the blood pH safe.

Enhanced Immune System

Using a ketogenic diet helps prevent the ageing of antioxidants and reduces inflammation of the gut, improving the immune system.

Reduced levels of cholesterol

The use of fewer carbs when you are on the keto diet helps lower blood cholesterol. This is due to increased lipolysis disease. This decreases LDL levels of cholesterol and raises HDL levels of cholesterol.

Appetite and cravings decreased.

Adopting the keto diet helps you reduce your calorie-rich food appetite and cravings. When you start to eat right, fulfilling and beneficial high-fat foods, your feelings of hunger will gradually begin to decline.

Weight Loss: Should You Indulge in Keto Snacks?

With many people now jumping on the "ketogenic diet," more and more people begin to question if this diet plan is for them. Even when you are not on a ketogenic diet, it would be hard to see keto food in your store now.

Marketers are conscious that the ketogenic diet does not seem to go where it was and start making satisfying snacks "ready to go."

Here are several points about keto items to bear in mind.

1. Calories Matter. First of all, take note that calories matter more than anything else here. So many individuals dive into eating keto snacks without caring too much about looking at calories. If you eat a snack that includes 400 calories, somewhere, you have to take part!

Compare this to the non-traditional keto snack like a 100-calorie apple, which is better for your weight loss plan? You can add peanut butter to the apple, and you'd still be less than 200 calories than the calories in the snack.

2. Does not actually mean "friendly weight loss." Also, note keto does not imply a friendly weight loss. Although several people use the ketogenic diet to lose weight, they still have to think of calories as stated. Some individuals use this diet for health reasons, and several of them are better promoted because they don't watch their calories too much.

It does not mean necessarily that it is intended to help you lose weight just because a product claims it is keto. The ketogenic diet is a low-carbs, fat diet that dramatically reduces your consumption of carbohydrate and removes fat.

3. Check Diet. Finally, take diet into account too. If the keto snack is as many refined and some of the high-carb snacks in their eating plans are to be substituted, they are also not all safe. The chocolate bar is really not a good idea, regardless of whether or not it is a keto bar. Don't lose common sense by merely seeing the word "keto."

You should be more prepared to decrypt the ads of keto items to ensure that they do not direct you away from your smart way of eating healthily if you consider these issues.

While the disorder can be complicated to handle, type 2 diabetes is not a condition in which you necessarily have to live. You can change your everyday routine simply and reduce both the weight and the blood sugar levels.

3 Ways Plan For Weight Loss

A fast weight loss program should not rely on calorie counts, or on fat grams forever. If you like to lose weight soon, then you must take steps aimed at rapid loss of weight instead of long-term loss of value. As it is essential to count calories for a long-term diet plan, a fast weight loss plan must use a few tricks to succeed.

1. Fasting. Some would simply not eat the most apparent and fast weight loss strategy. There are also several dangerous flags that rise when you think of fasting. However, fasting can be done in a healthy way, and there are many health practitioners who still recommend that the system is cleaned up regularly quickly. Remember that much of the weight that you lose is water weight and fast should be performed only

for a limited period of time and should be carried out according to proper directives for a specific form of fasting procedure that you are pursuing. You will still take some liquid and eat plenty of vitamins in balanced fasting routines. This can be a quick weight loss scheme, but it can be very challenging, and a lot of the weight you lose is water.

2. Carb Quick. This easy weight loss plan is a little better than the whole fast because, besides water weight loss, you lose more fat. In turn, you cut out all carbohydrates from your diet and only eat protein and fat in combination. It typically lasts 2 to 5 days before your body turns over and starts using fat, since it is a primary source of energy, so your body naturally burns both your fat and your own fat. After the five or sixth day (for 1-2 days), re-load carbohydrates and then restart carbohydrate for another five days. The explanation of why this can be considered a simple weight loss plan is because most people experience immediate results with carb fast out of all diets out there. A search under "keto diet" should be performed to learn the exact procedures for executing this quick weight loss plan safely and efficiently.

3. Take supplements! Losing weight in the shortest possible period requires some external support. The body can't naturally burn fat alone that fast. You should take the right supplements. Many are called fat blockers or binders or burners. Others are certainly less effective than others, and it is also always interesting to find out what compounds function safely and efficiently for your fast weight loss plan. And continuously pursue natural products as your first choice as they exist and have many advantages, including being the ideal addition to your rapid weight loss plan!

Keto and Low-Carb Recipe Ideas

You can still eat pizza on a keto diet, but imagination is required. I order a thin-crowned pizza when I dine out, then take my fork and slip all the toppings away. It helps order a pizza with several toppings. If you order a deep-dish pizza, you have very little left to eat.

As is the case for most food choices on keto, you make the best pizza. Try the low-carbs pizza crust recipe and use these toppings:

Mexican pizza — Top with taco or chicken, or regular (low carb) sauce or enchilada sauce. Add a little salsa, chopped onions, jalapeno chopped peppers, and some spicy sauce (the lowest in carbs for Taco Bell). Add chopped cilantro to any extra spice. And after baking, top with sliced avocado.

Greek pizza-sauce, red onions, feta, olives and artichoke hearts, how about this?

Buffalo chicken Pizza-I've been excited to discover Frank's low-carb red-hot buffalo wing sauce. If you like spicy, hot or sweet, you can make a hot pizza using grilled chicken, some ointments, crumbled blue cheese and a buffalo sauce. Don't forget to drizzle over the top of a little blue cheese.

Indian Pizza-There is a small nearby pizza-specific restaurant that gave me the idea to make my own. If you want to make this delicious choice, you can add some veggies to a packaged Indian food savoring on top of the low-carbs crust. If you're going to start with the traditional Indian spices from the scratch season, including curry powder, masala, cumin and any other spicy Indian seasoning, you might imagine. If needed, add vegetables.

Alfredo Pizza-Use Alfredo sauce to eat or only scoop some of it out of a container. Top with parsley and chicken, plus garlic, shrimp, tomatoes from Roma and, if you like, extra parmesan.

Of course, all of the standard pizza options are available:

Meat lovers, whatever you want, pepperoni, sausage, bacon, pork. These are shallow low carbs options.

Fans of Veggie- Onions, Mushrooms, tomatoes, all sorts of artichoke, peppers. It'll taste fantastic.

Three (or four or five) cheese pizza — Try, in addition to or in place, the usually shredded mozzarella, feta cheese, blue cheese, cream cheese and goat cheese, or some other tangy mozzarella. (Remember that there are several low-carbs crusts made of cheese too. Maybe you'd like to overdo it!)

Once you have a healthy low carbs crust, the overarching ideas are infinite. Keto dieters have many choices. Your imagination is the only limit.

The ketogenic diet is the right choice for those looking to lose weight.

Ketogenic Diets For Type 2 Diabetes Management

Through the keto diet, the body converts fat into energy instead of sugar. Ketones are a process by-product.

Diabetes has been treated with ketogenic diets over the years. One purpose was to cure diabetes at the source by reducing carbohydrate consumption, which in turn decreases the need for insulin,that minimizes insulin resistance or metabolic syndrome. This can increase blood glucose (sugar) levels by a ketogenic diet while simultaneously reducing the need for insulin. This view reflects a much better and productive strategy for keto diets than for insulin to combat high carbohydrate intake.

In reality, a keto diet is a very restrictive diet. For example, in the classical Keto diet, approximately 80% of caloric demand is extracted from fat and 20% from proteins and carbohydrates. This is a marked divergence from the standard in which the body uses energy from sugar provided by carbohydrate digestion but is forced to use fat by significantly restricting carbohydrates.

The ketogenic diet calls for balanced food consumption from beneficial fats, such as grass butter, cocoa oil, organic grassy eggs, avocados, salmon, cottage cheese, avocados, almond kinds of butter and crude nuts (rough pecans and macadamia). Ketogenic people avoid all types of bread, flour, rice, pasta, potatoes, starchy food and dairy foods. The diet has a low content of vitamins, minerals and nutrients and different extra treatment.

Low carbohydrate diet is also prescribed for people with type 2 since carbohydrates transform to blood sugar that spikes blood sugar in large amounts. For a diabetic who already has elevated blood sugar, it is like courting the possibility of consuming different foods generating sugar. Some patients may experience lowered blood sugar by switching the emphasis from sugar to fat.

Changing the primary main energy source of the body from carbohydrates to fat leaves ketones in the blood behind the fat metabolism by-product. This may be risky individual train diabetic patients as the growth of ketones may establish risk for diabetic ketoacidosis (DKA). DKA is a medical emergency that needs a physician immediately. DKA symptoms consistently include dry mouth, high blood sugar, nausea, polyuria, the fruit-like odor and trouble breathing. Diabetic coma can be caused by complications.

Conclusion

The ketogenic diet is a perfect choice for many people for weight loss. It is very different and enables a person on a diet to consume a diet consisting of foods you would not expect.

If you eat very low carbohydrates, the body becomes ketose. What this implies is that the body burns energy with fat. How much glucose do you need to eat to get ketosis? Well, it differs from one person to another, but it's a safe bet to remain below 25 net carbs. Some would say that you should stay under ten net carbs while you are in the 'induction stage,' when you are in ketosis.

Net carbs are carbs quantity you consume less dietary fiber. If you eat 35 g of net carbs and 13 g of dietary fiber per day, your net carbs will be 22 per day. Simple enough, right?

Well, some people talk of their enhanced mental clarity while they are on a diet. Another advantage is an improvement in energy. Another is a diminishing appetite.

Something one needs to think about when doing a ketogenic diet is called ketogenic flu. Not everyone will feel this, but this can be hard to accomplish.

Sounds like a diet you'd like to be interested in, so what are you waiting for? Dive head in keto today.